D0190633

The Coumadin® (Warfarin) Help Book

*A Guide to Anticoagulation Therapy
to Prevent and Manage Strokes,
Heart Attacks, and
Other Vascular Disorders*

Diana M. Schneider, Ph.D.

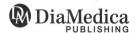
DiaMedica
PUBLISHING

DiaMedica Publishing, 150 East 61st Street, New York, NY 10065

Visit our website at www.diamedicapub.com

ISBN: 978-0-9793564-2-1

Note to Readers

This book is not a substitute for medical advice and assistance. Coumadin® and warfarin have the potential to cause serious side effects, such that a "Black-Box Warning" about them is now included with the prescribing information. The judgment of individual physicians and other medical specialists who know you and manage your treatment is essential. Although the information in this book was developed to help you better understand and manage your anticoagulant therapy, it is not intended to replace your own physician's medical advice.

Trademarked names are used throughout this book. Rather than note the trademark symbol after every occurrence of a trademarked name, we use names in an editorial fashion only, and to the benefit of the trademark owner, with no intention of infringement of the trademark. The symbol appears whenever a trademarked name is used in the title of a chapter, and for its first use within each chapter. Wherever such designations appear in this book, they have been printed with initial Caps, as in Coumadin®.

Editor: Jessica Bryan
Designed and typeset by: TypeWriting

To John, for everything

Acknowledgments

I am deeply grateful to the friends, colleagues, and health care professionals who took the time to read the draft manuscript of this book and who made many valuable suggestions. Special thanks to Gary Liska, James W. Miller, M.D., Vivien Jean Ang, N.P., Nelly Vega-Woo, N.P., Ron Franz, and Maggie Lichtenberg.

Contents

Introduction

YOU ARE READING THIS BOOK because you, a family member, or a friend needs to take either Coumadin® or its generic form, warfarin. These medications are *oral* (taken by mouth) *anticoagulants* (preventing blood clotting)—also called "blood thinners." They do not in fact "thin" the blood, but instead slow its ability to clot by decreasing the activity of clotting factors produced by the liver.

You might be finding that it is difficult to maintain your blood clotting time within the therapeutically effective range (as measured by the "INR"), resulting in the need for frequent monitoring and dosage adjustment. You might have read the package insert for your medication, and perhaps done a bit of reading on the Internet. If so, you are probably concerned about possible side effects of anticoagulants, as well as what appear to be significant restrictions on what you can eat and potential problems with other medications.

You are most definitely not alone! Between two and three million Americans now take Coumadin or warfarin, and 300,000 to 500,000 people start on these drugs every year as a result of the conditions discussed in Chapter 3.

These are not medications that should be taken casually. Coumadin and warfarin are responsible for 15 percent of all

What Is an INR?

The blood test that measures the time it takes your blood to clot is called the *prothrombin time* or PT. However, the term you will most often hear is *International Normalized Ratio* or INR. We repeatedly mention the INR throughout this book, because it is the key to maintaining your clotting levels in the desired range. The INR measures clotting time in a standardized way that takes into account differences in age, gender, and testing method. The test can be performed in your doctor's office, a monitoring clinic, or at home, depending on your specific needs. It involves either a simple finger prick or a blood draw, depending on where you have the test done.

serious adverse drug reactions in the United States each year, and five of the ten most serious drug interactions in older individuals occur with these oral anticoagulants. The U.S. Food and Drug Administration (FDA) has issued a "Black-Box Warning," to be included on the medication insert that comes with each prescription, indicating that the drug can cause "major" or "fatal" bleeding, which is most likely to occur during the starting period or at higher doses. Risk factors for bleeding include age 65 or over; a high intensity of anticoagulation (an INR greater than 4); highly variable INRs; a history of gastrointestinal bleeding, hypertension, cerebrovascular disease, serious heart disease, anemia, malignancy, trauma, or renal insufficiency; the need to take other medications; and a long duration of therapy. The warning recommends frequent INR monitoring, careful dose adjustment to the desired range, and a shorter duration of therapy when possible.

Despite this, with appropriate care and attention, the vast majority of people taking Coumadin or warfarin do so successfully, without any adverse effects. To be sure that you stay in this majority, it is necessary to take a few basic precautions. These primarily involve taking reasonable care to maintain a consistent diet, and being aware of what types of medications can cause problems when taken with your oral anticoagulant. This book was developed to help you do just that.

It is divided into three sections. Section I discusses the basics—what an anticoagulant is, why controlling clotting is important, the consequences of abnormal clot formation, and common conditions that cause clots to form. Section II focuses on successful anticoagulation management, with chapters on how anticoagulants should be taken, monitoring, side effects, the importance of a consistent diet, how drugs and supplements affect anticoagulants, and how other medical conditions can affect coagulation management. Section III discusses general health concerns and managing your therapy when away from home. A detailed list of resources will lead you to additional helpful information.

Much of the information in this book is available on the Internet. However, doing a detailed search and evaluating information from multiple sources is not what anyone wants to do when a major medical issue occurs without warning. This book will get you started, and point you in the right direction for getting additional information and answering specific questions when you have the time to do so.

From the Author:
How to Use This Book

I'VE BEEN IN PUBLISHING for over 30 years, and developed and published about 600 books during that time. But, until now, I've never written one. Why now, and why a book on Coumadin®/warfarin?

About five years ago, I began to notice that I was extremely out of breath while climbing the subway stairs (I live in Manhattan and that's my main mode of getting around town). Since I was going to my health club four or five times a week, this didn't make sense to me. At first, my internist thought my problem was probably nothing major, although an echocardiogram showed that the right side of my heart was enlarged. Eventually, after a series of pulmonary and cardiac tests, we discovered that I had been born with a *septal defect*, an opening between the two *atria*—the upper chambers of the heart. This is basically a mild version of the "blue baby" syndrome that you might have heard about in the past—many or most of these defects are now detected early and repaired in infancy or childhood.

This condition was responsible for my enlarged heart, and I learned that it was associated with a seriously increased risk of stroke. As my heart had no other abnormalities, I appeared to be a good candidate for a relatively new surgical technique. This was a "minimally invasive" procedure to insert a device that would close the opening. It involved only small incisions in the groin area, and was similar to the relatively common procedure of inserting a *stent* to open blood vessels that have developed atherosclerotic plaques, in order to prevent a heart attack.

The procedure was successfully accomplished; I was in the hospital overnight, and returned to work a few days later. Miracle of modern surgery, for sure! I went on Coumadin therapy, with the idea that I would need it for about three months until the device in my heart was covered with normal tissue and no longer a potential site of clot formation. Unfortunately, a month later, I had a mild stroke. I was lucky—I have only a slight loss of vision as a result, which is a nuisance but not more than that. My cardiologist was sure that I had developed an *atrial fibrillation*—a type of *arrhythmia* or abnormal heart rhythm. It could not be detected while I was in the hospital but—on a routine visit—there it was. Bad luck, indeed!

I soon found that managing Coumadin was going to take some time and effort. For example, when I thought I was going to be on the drug for only a few months, I just gave up eating leafy greens—the major source of vitamin K, which counteracts the effect of Coumadin or warfarin, and is discussed in detail later in this book. This was not a good choice for the long run, so my Coumadin/warfarin clinic nurse and I adjusted my dosage to accommodate one serving of leafy greens or a green vegetable each day. I also found out that I needed to avoid the common pain medications ibuprofen and aspirin. Based on this, I modified both my diet and medications. Most importantly, I learned that the key factors in maintaining my level of clotting in the appropriate range, as measured by the INR, are *consistency* and *moderation*. These important concepts are major themes of this book. You can accommodate *any* change in your diet, medications, or lifestyle—within reason of course—by understanding how to take some straightforward and simple precautions.

I was surprised to find out how many people use Coumadin or its generic version, warfarin. Most of the people I spoke with had trouble keeping their levels steady. Instead of the four- to six-week interval between testing that I needed, they had to be tested weekly or biweekly, with their INR going up and down in seemingly random fashion. Of course, it wasn't really random at all. Instead of the good and careful advice and information I had received, often no one had told them about the simple steps they needed to take and—amazing to me—quite often no one had even explained how diet and medications could affect their INR.

Still others had the opposite experience. Either they were given the information they needed but did not really understand it, or they found it so overwhelming and complicated that they stopped trying to manage their levels. This was especially true if they were led to believe that they needed to monitor their food intake so carefully that practically every mouthful needed to be analyzed for its vitamin K content.

When I began to search for information about these oral anticoagulants, I found that a lot of material is available on the Internet, but it is widely scattered and of variable reliability. More importantly, it is often conflicting and confusing. As a medical publisher, I am often asked for advice by friends and family, and I've learned to refer them to selected information from reliable medical organizations and U.S. government sources. The material I began to accumulate formed the basis of this book, and I've included a detailed Resources section to help you search for additional information that will be helpful in your journey to successfully managing your medication.

This book was written so that it can be read either start-to-finish or on an as-needed basis. If you are just beginning to take Coumadin or warfarin, read it through completely, and then return to the appropriate sections when you have questions or problems. If you already have experience with managing your anticoagulant, you might want to read specific sections and use the Resources section to expand your knowledge about your medication.

The following brief overview will help you start managing your Coumadin or warfarin. Each topic is discussed in detail later in the book.

General Guidelines for Successfully Managing Coumadin and Warfarin

These guidelines will be discussed in greater detail in subsequent chapters, but this brief summary will help you "get up to speed" quickly on some of the major issues you need to be concerned about.

- ▶ Do not take aspirin or other *nonsteroidal anti-inflammatory drugs* (NSAIDs) unless your doctor has told you it is safe to do so and your medication is adjusted, if needed. These drugs can affect blood clotting and can cause serious bleeding in your stomach or intestines (see Chapter 8). NSAIDs include aspirin, ibuprofen (Motrin®, Advil®), naproxen (Aleve®, Naprosyn®), celecoxib (Celebrex®), and diclofenac (Voltaren®).
- ▶ Check with your physician or nurse before taking any new medication to find out if the new drug might affect coagulation and whether you need to modify your dosage of Coumadin or warfarin, or have additional INR testing done while you are tak-

ing the drug (See Chapter 8). For example, sulfa drugs and a wide variety of commonly used antibiotics can result in your needing to reduce your anticoagulant dose by as much as 50 percent. If not monitored properly—which includes your own checks for signs of bleeding, such as excessive bruising—you run the risk of excessive bleeding.

▶ Avoid sudden changes in your diet, especially the amounts of vitamin K–containing leafy green vegetables and other foods that contain large amounts of this vitamin. As discussed in Chapter 1, vitamin K decreases the effects of Coumadin and warfarin. Do not change the amount of these foods in your diet without first talking to your health care provider.

▶ Be sure to talk to your physician or nurse before you attempt to lose or gain weight. If, for example, you want to lose any substantial weight, you might need to gradually reduce the amount of anticoagulant medication to compensate for a smaller body mass.

▶ Drink alcohol only in moderation. Like the NSAIDs, alcohol can increase blood levels of Coumadin or warfarin. Although some sources suggest that alcohol should be avoided completely, moderation is probably reasonable for most people—generally defined as no more than two drinks each day. Excessive drinking can lead to liver damage, which can have major effects on the blood-clotting system.

▶ Avoid smoking cigarettes or chewing tobacco. Besides their other health effects—and the increasing lack of acceptance of these unpleasant habits—tobacco can alter the blood levels of your oral anticoagulant.

▶ Avoid hazardous activities and sports that might lead to injury or broken skin, as well as activities such as working on ladders that can result in falls. If you currently have an exercise routine that involves physical contact or has the potential for serious injury, speak with your physician about safety issues. Also, if you are changing your exercise pattern or planning to start one, speak to your physician prior to beginning any new activities.

▶ You might find it useful to keep one or two "hemostatic" gauze pads in your purse or wallet, which stop bleeding almost instantly (see Resources).

Section I

The Basics: Why Anticoagulation Is Necessary

THIS SECTION PROVIDES background information on three topics: the process of blood clotting and how an anticoagulant is used to prevent unwanted clotting; the serious medical consequences of clot formation, including strokes, heart attacks, and pulmonary embolisms; and a background discussion of the common medical conditions that cause dangerous clots to form.

If you are an experienced user of Coumadin® or warfarin—and are knowledgeable about the cause of the condition that requires you to use an oral anticoagulant medication—you might wish to proceed directly to Section II.

What Is an Anticoagulant, and Why Is Controlling Blood Clotting So Important?

A BLOOD CLOT IS the gelatinous mass that normally forms whenever we experience any type of cut or injury, and normal blood clotting is essential to life. However, blood clots also can develop as the result of a number of medical conditions that involve the heart, lungs, and vascular system. When they form at the wrong time and in the wrong place, clots can lead to a heart attack, stroke, or pulmonary embolism, so it is extremely important that they be prevented.

When clots form at the wrong time and in the wrong place, they can lead to a heart attack, stroke, or pulmonary embolism.

Anti means against, and *coagulant* refers to blood clotting, so an *anticoagulant* helps to prevent clots from forming in the blood. Coumadin® and generic warfarin are long-acting oral anticoagulants, as distinct from rapid- and short-acting anticoagulants that must be injected.

Before we can discuss the conditions that lead to unwanted clot formation, the serious conditions that result, and how anticoagulants work, you need to understand a bit about the *circulatory system* and the process of *blood clotting*.

THE CIRCULATORY SYSTEM

Figure 1.1 shows the pathway that blood takes through the circulatory system, which includes the heart, lungs, and blood vessels. The system is essentially a large double loop—one between the heart and lungs, and one involving the heart and general circulation. It provides oxygenated blood to the tissues of the body, and then returns this blood to the heart when it is depleted of oxygen, and the cycle begins again.

The right side of this diagram includes the left side of the heart (remember, you are looking at this "head on") and the arterial system that delivers blood to all the tissues of the body, called the *systemic* circulation. The blood it contains has been provided with oxygen by the lungs. After oxygen is removed from the arterial part of the system by the tissues of the body, it enters the venous system. This blood enters the right side of the heart, where it is pumped to the lungs to be oxygenated. It then enters the left side of the heart to be once again pumped into the arterial system, repeating the cycle. This pumping system depends on a complex system of nerves that runs throughout the heart, causing its muscles to contract in just the right sequence to allow for smooth and continuous pumping.

This smoothly functioning system can develop a number of problems, many of which result in an increased tendency to form clots. Anticoagulants are prescribed for people who are at increased risk for developing harmful blood clots and for those who have already experienced a problem due to clots.

Head and Arms

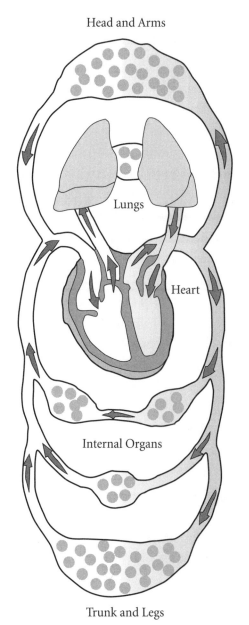

Lungs

Heart

Internal Organs

Trunk and Legs

FIGURE 1.1 THIS DIAGRAM OF THE CIRCULATORY SYSTEM SHOWS HOW BLOOD TRAVELS FROM THE HEART TO THE LUNGS AND THEN TO THE INTERNAL ORGANS, HEAD, AND EXTREMITY.

Individuals at risk for developing clots include people who have the irregular heart rhythm called *atrial fibrillation* (AF), a mechanical heart valve, and those with disorders of the clotting system itself. People with a history of developing harmful clots have experienced a stroke, a heart attack, a clot that traveled to the lung (pulmonary embolism or PE), or a blood clot in the leg (deep venous thrombosis or DVT).

The number of people who take the anticoagulant medications Coumadin or warfarin has increased rapidly, because the number of conditions for which they have been shown to be effective has increased. When clots do occur, they reduce blood flow to the organs whose blood supply is provided by the vessel in which the clot formed. A stroke results when a blood vessel leading to a portion of the brain is blocked; a heart attack occurs when a blood vessel leading to the heart is blocked; and a pulmonary embolus occurs when a clot formed in the right side of the heart lodges in the lungs.

WHAT CONTROLS BLOOD CLOTTING?

Blood clotting after a cut or injury is essential to life. The process by which clotting occurs is called *coagulation*, and the total process of blood clotting followed by the clot dissolving and repair of the injured tissue is termed *hemostasis*.

Hemostasis consists of four steps:

▶ The blood vessels in the area of the injury constrict, limiting blood flow to the area that has been injured.

▶ *Platelets* (cells that circulate in the blood) are activated by a substance called *thrombin*, which is released when an injury occurs. The platelets then migrate into the area of injury, where they form a loose plug. These platelets then clump by binding to *collagen*, which is released by damaged blood vessels in the injured area. The platelets then release additional substances that are important for coagulation.

▶ To stabilize the initially loose platelet plug, a *fibrin mesh* (the clot) forms around and within the plug.

▶ Finally, when sufficient healing has occurred, the clot dissolves and normal blood flow to the injured area can resume.

The process of clot formation involves a group of proteins called *clotting factors*, which are made in the liver. The pathway through which clotting occurs—the *coagulation cascade*—is shown schematically in Figure 1.2. It is not necessary to understand the details of this complex process, only that Coumadin or warfarin affects the activity of some of the proteins involved, and that this in turn prevents the formation of clots at the wrong time and in the wrong place. The drugs do so by inhibiting the activity of the vitamin K–dependent clotting factors involved in the clotting cascade. The involvement of so many substances and the complexity of the clotting cascade are the reasons why the system is so sensitive to the content of vitamin K in your diet, and why it can be difficult to maintain a constant level of clotting when using an anticoagulant.

How Is Vitamin K Involved in the Clotting Process?

Vitamins are nutrients that are required in very small amounts in order for essential metabolic reactions to occur in the body.

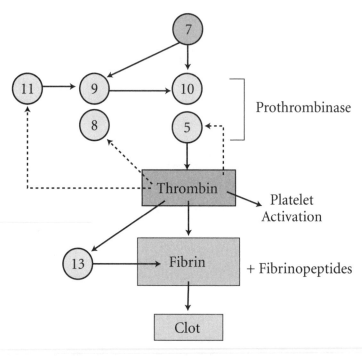

FIGURE 1.2 THE COAGULATION CASCADE. THE NUMBERS REFER TO CLOTTING FACTORS.

All vitamins act as *catalysts* in chemical reactions that are essential to life. In this role, they bind to enzymes and are termed *cofactors*. The "K" in vitamin K is from the Danish word for coagulation, "koagulering," in honor of the Danish scientist who discovered it.

Vitamin K is an essential cofactor for the action of an enzyme that allows substances needed in the clotting pathway to bind calcium, without which clotting cannot occur. Of particular importance is its role in the synthesis of *prothrombin* in the liver. Remember, your regular blood tests while on Coumadin measure "prothrombin time" or PT; the INR is a normalized version of this measurement. You can see from Figure 1.2 that *prothrombin* and its derivative molecule *throm-*

bin are central components in the clotting process, so your INR actually measures the activity of this essential component of the clotting process.

Coumadin and warfarin block the availability of vitamin K and limit production of the clotting factors. As a result, it takes longer for the blood to clot.

The interaction between vitamin K and anticoagulants is competitive in nature. The more vitamin K in the diet, the less effective Coumadin or warfarin becomes. However, as long as your diet remains constant with respect to vitamin K, the dose of anticoagulant can be adjusted to overcome this effect.

Only small amounts of vitamin K are stored in the body, and it must be constantly replenished through the diet. Coumadin and warfarin prevent its reuse, essentially causing a deficiency of the vitamin and thus inhibiting clot formation. The medication does this by inhibiting two important chemical reactions in the clotting system. So, a sort of "push–pull" interaction occurs between the anticoagulant medication and vitamin K. The trick is to keep them in balance, which you probably already know since you are reading this book!

Sources of Vitamin K

There are actually two sources of vitamin K. One—called *vitamin K1*—is probably already familiar to you because of the need to maintain a constant level of leafy greens and other vitamin K–containing foods in your diet. The other—*vitamin K2*—is made by bacteria in the gut. The K2 form can be affected by illnesses such as influenza (the "flu"), which can deplete the level of these helpful bacteria. Vitamin K1 is manufactured for medicinal use as Mephyton®, and is occasionally used to rapidly decrease the rate of clotting should your INR become extremely high or should you need emergency surgery.

Never try to manage your vitamin K levels yourself with herbal versions of vitamin K—they are not regulated for purity or consistency of content, and you need your physician's or nurse's assistance if your INR is seriously increased or you are in need of surgery.

The next two chapters discuss what happens when clots form in the vascular system, and what conditions can lead to clot formation.

2

The Consequences of Abnormal Clot Formation: Stroke, Heart Attacks, and More

WHEN CLOTS FORM anywhere in the blood vessels of the vascular system, they can break away from the vessel wall and travel through the vascular system. Eventually, they lodge in blood vessels that are smaller than the size of the clot. Most often, this means the brain, heart tissue, or lungs, where they cause strokes, heart attacks, or pulmonary emboli. This can be fatal, or it can result in significant disability. What are these conditions, and why is it so important to do everything possible to avoid them?

STROKE

Stroke is the third largest cause of death annually in the United States, after heart disease and cancer, and the leading cause of adult disability. Over 5 million Americans have survived a stroke. Worldwide, approximately 10 percent of all deaths are due to stroke. The Centers for Disease Control puts the number of new or recurrent strokes at about 700,000 each year, and the annual number of deaths at 150,000.

Stroke is the third largest cause of death annually in the United States, and the leading cause of adult disability.

The term *stroke,* also referred to as a *cerebrovascular accident* (CVA), is used for any rapid loss of brain function that occurs as the result of a problem in the vessels that supply blood to the brain. This can be due either to *ischemia*—a lack of blood supply and oxygen caused by a blood clot, or to a *hemorrhage*—a leakage of blood from these vessels. Eighty percent of all strokes are of the ischemic type; 20 percent are hemorrhagic.

Both types of stroke are important for people who take Coumadin® or warfarin. The most common reason for taking these anticoagulants is to prevent the development of a blood clot that can cause an ischemic stroke by blocking a blood vessel. They are prescribed to people at high risk for developing blood clots, and to those who have already experienced a stroke.

Bleeding from a hemorrhagic stroke is one of the most dangerous consequences of too high a level of anticoagulant and a seriously increased INR.

Maintaining the INR in the desired therapeutic range is critical to avoiding both problems. The risk of stroke doubles as the INR decreases from 2.0 to 1.7 in people with atrial fibrillation (AF) whose target range INR is 2.0 to 3.0, and it more than doubles again if the INR is reduced to 1.4.

Conversely, bleeding from a hemorrhagic stroke is one of the most dangerous consequences of too high a level of anticoagulant and a seriously increased INR. To put "seriously increased" into perspective, an INR of 4.0 nearly doubles the risk of a bleeding incident over that with an INR of 3.0 or less—and the risk of a serious bleed increases nearly sevenfold with an INR of over 6.0.

High-risk cardiac causes of ischemic stroke include AF, rheumatic disease of the mitral or aortic valve, and artificial heart valves. In people who have AF without any damage to the heart valves, anticoagulation can reduce the risk of stroke by 60 percent.

A major focus in treating people with these conditions is called *secondary prevention*—actions that can be taken to reduce the risk of a stroke in those who already have diseases or risk factors that are known to cause stroke, as well as in people who have already had one or more strokes. Medication or drug therapy is the most common method of stroke prevention. Aspirin—usually low-dose or "baby" aspirin—is often recommended. People with abnormalities of the heart that put them at risk for developing an ischemic stroke, or who have already had one, often require anticoagulation with medications such as Coumadin or warfarin.

See the Resources at the end of this book for information on websites that have detailed information about stroke.

HEART ATTACKS

Over 25 million people in the United States have heart disease, and nearly a million people have a heart attack—an *acute myocardial infarction*—each year. Heart disease is the leading cause of death in the United States—one in five deaths, or over 650,000 annually. Worldwide, over 12 percent of deaths are due to ischemic heart disease.

A heart attack occurs when the blood supply to the heart is interrupted. A blood clot is the most common cause of a blocked coronary artery. Usually, the artery is already partially narrowed by an *atherosclerotic plaque.* This can rupture or tear, narrowing the artery still further and making blockage by a clot more likely. The ruptured plaque material reduces the flow of blood through the artery, and it also releases substances that make platelets stickier, further encouraging clots to form. The resulting *ischemia* or oxygen shortage causes damage and potential death of heart tissue. One of the more important risk factors for a heart attack is an *arrhythmia,* one of the reasons that AF is normally treated with an oral anticoagulant.

Following a heart attack, the injured heart tissue conducts electrical impulses more slowly than normal heart tissue. The imbalance between normal conduction in the undamaged tissue and slowed conduction in the damaged area is believed to be the cause of many of the arrhythmias that occur following a heart attack. The most serious of these is *ventricular fibrillation,* an extremely fast and chaotic heart rhythm that is the leading cause of sudden cardiac death.

A substantial number of people who have had a heart attack subsequently experience clot formation in the left ventricle, as the result of damaged heart tissue. These clots, or parts of them, can break off and travel through the bloodstream; if they travel to the brain, they will cause a stroke.

Anticoagulants are commonly prescribed to help prevent clot formation after a heart attack, especially if the heart attack was massive, or if areas of the heart are not beating well. An anticoagulant is usually taken for three to six months after a heart attack, often maintaining the INR at 2.5 to 3.5.

For more detailed information about myocardial infarction, see the Resources section at the end of this book.

VENOUS THROMBOEMBOLISM: DEEP VEIN THROMBOSIS AND PULMONARY EMBOLISM

An estimated 2 million people in the United States develop a *venous thromboembolism* (VTE) each year. About 600,000 are hospitalized, and 60,000 die.

The term VTE refers both to *deep vein thrombosis* (DVT) and pulmonary embolism (PE). A *venous thrombosis* is a blood clot that forms in the venous system, most commonly in the legs. It can cause calf pain and tenderness, sometimes accompanied by redness, warmth, and swelling of the leg. However, some people are not aware of any symptoms.

Although it can occur in young, otherwise healthy adults, DVT most frequently occurs following trauma, major surgery, prolonged immobility (including airline travel), or in people who have a clotting disorder. Other risk factors include obesity, smoking, and hypertension. Chronic medical conditions such as heart failure and cancer, as well as oral contraceptives and hormone replacement therapy (HRT), also increase the risk of DVT. Any risk factor for DVT also increases the risk that the venous clot will dislodge and migrate to the lung circulation. This happens in up to 15 percent of all DVTs.

Pulmonary embolism most often occurs when one or more of these dislodged clots lodges in the pulmonary artery or one of its branches, causing a partial or complete obstruction of blood flow to a portion of lung tissue. Symptoms can include the sudden onset of shortness of breath, rapid breathing, chest pain, and coughing. More severe cases might be associated with a bluish discoloration, usually of the lips and fingers (cyanosis), collapse, and circulatory instability. About 15 percent of all cases of sudden death are attributable to PE.

The duration of anticoagulant therapy following a VTE varies, depending on whether it is the first time a clot has occurred or if they have occurred previously, the location of the clot(s), and any medical conditions that increase your chances of subsequent clot formation. However, you will require anticoagulant therapy for a minimum of three to six months.

In 2004, the American College of Chest Physicians updated its recommendations for the optimal therapeutic ranges for oral anticoagulation, with an INR "target range" of 2.0 to 3.0 for most indications. The exceptions include patients with some types of mechanical heart valves and post–myocardial infarction, for which a higher INR range is suggested (2.5–3.5). The suggested duration of therapy varies, from several months after an episode—such as a first PE or certain types of cardiac surgery—to lifelong therapy for ongoing AF.

3

Common Conditions That
Cause Clots to Form

ATRIAL FIBRILLATION

ATRIAL FIBRILLATION (AF) is the most common form of arrhythmia, a disruption of the normal heart rhythm. It affects approximately 2.2 million people in the United States alone, including about 4 percent of all people over age 60, and almost 10 percent of those over 80. This condition involves an irregular, rapid contraction of the left and right *atria*—the top chambers of the heart (Figure 3.1). The atria normally beat smoothly in a rhythm with the *ventricles*—the lower chambers of the heart— allowing for the smooth movement of blood throughout the system, as discussed in Chapter 1. In AF, this rhythm is disrupted—hence the term *arrhythmia*. The atria might beat several hundred times per minute, which can have the effect of raising the heart rate from the normal level of 60 to 100 beats each minute to as high as 180

Atrial fibrillation (AF) is the most common form of arrhythmia, a disruption of the normal heart rhythm.

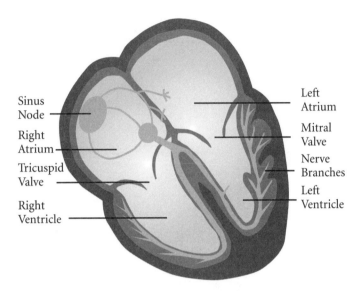

Sinus Node

Right Atrium

Tricuspid Valve

Right Ventricle

Left Atrium

Mitral Valve

Nerve Branches

Left Ventricle

FIGURE 3.1 THIS SIMPLIFIED DIAGRAM OF THE HEART SHOWS THE ATRIA AND VENTRICLES, THE MAJOR VALVES BETWEEN THEM, AND THE ELECTRICAL SYSTEM THAT CONTROLS ITS SMOOTH FUNCTIONING.

beats per minute; however, many people do not experience any significant increase in pulse rate. Atrial fibrillation makes it difficult for the left atrium to empty blood into the left ventricle, which pumps it to the rest of the body. The result is that the blood supply to the body is insufficient, causing shortness of breath and other symptoms.

Atrial fibrillation can occur in otherwise healthy individuals. But, in most cases, it is associated with an underlying heart condition or, occasionally, with thyroid disorders. For example, I take Coumadin® because AF developed as the result of a distortion of the normal heart structure and underlying electrical conduction system following repair of a birth defect I had lived with all my life.

Some people with AF experience no symptoms, or only minor ones. Others experience a range of symptoms that might include *palpitations*, during which they feel the rapid beating of their heart; fatigue; dizziness; shortness of breath; and chest pain. As many as 70 percent of people with AF are not aware of any symptoms; the condition is found on a physician's examination, often for an unrelated matter. It is important to recognize the symptoms of AF, so that you can discuss them with your doctor. Even if you are not bothered by your AF, it is extremely important to determine whether it should be treated with anticoagulant therapy. Atrial fibrillation increases the risk of stroke dramatically—*one of every six strokes occurs in a person who has AF*. These numbers are huge; there are almost 900,000 hospital discharges every year after stroke, and about 150,000 deaths.

These strokes occur because blood clots form in the left atrium as the result of blood not moving smoothly through the system. These clots then break free and lodge in an artery of the brain, cutting off blood supply to the area supplied by that blood vessel.

Sometimes, the normal rhythm of the heart can be restored either by stimulating the electrical system of the heart—a procedure called *cardioversion* or *electrocardioversion*, or by *cauterizing* (burning out) the small area of the electrical system that is responsible for an arrhythmia. Some people with AF are good candidates for medications that can restore normal heart rhythm or slow the heart rate. If these procedures are not appropriate for you, or they have been tried and failed, you may need to remain on an anticoagulant, probably for the rest of your life. This will depend on your particular situation, and recommendations may change based on new information. For example, people under age 65 who have no other problems besides an arrhythmia and do not have structural heart disease may not need to take an oral anticoagulant, while people over age 65 and younger individuals who have structural heart abnormalities most probably will.

Like me, you might also need to take aspirin, because this combination is considered to provide more protection than Coumadin or warfarin alone in some people. Aspirin has a different type of effect than the oral anticoagulant medications; it affects the "stickiness" of blood platelets but not the clotting cascade.

PROSTHETIC HEART VALVES

People who have mechanical prosthetic valves are often treated with a combination of aspirin and an oral anticoagulant. This condition is associated with a higher risk of clot formation than many of the other conditions treated with anticoagulants, and the INR is often maintained in the 2.5 to 3.5 range because of this level of risk. This range is recommended by the American College of Chest Physicians for most patients with mechanical prosthetic valves. Individuals with *bioprosthetic* heart valves—made of human or animal tissue—and low-risk patients with bileaflet mechanical valves such as the St. Jude Medical device may not need to take Coumadin or warfarin.

The combination of low-dose aspirin and high-intensity anticoagulant

In people with prosthetic heart valves, the combination of low-dose aspirin and high-intensity anticoagulant therapy appears to be associated with a statistically significant reduction in overall mortality, including deaths from cardiovascular disease and stroke.

therapy appears to be associated with a statistically significant reduction in overall mortality, including deaths from cardio-vascular disease and stroke. However, this significant benefit can be associated with an increase in minor bleeding problems and a very slight trend toward an increase in major bleeding problems. Your physician will weigh the risks and benefits of this combined therapy before making a decision about recommending this approach.

OTHER INDICATIONS FOR ORAL ANTICOAGULANTS

Other conditions that are widely accepted to be good candidates for anticoagulant therapy have not been as well studied as AF or valve replacement. These include people with congestive heart failure, people who have valvular heart disease that is associated with AF, and some people who have mitral valve problems. All of these carry a high risk of clot formation. Anticoagulation is also indicated for people who have had one or more episodes of thromboembolism due to unknown causes. Anticoagulants are not presently indicated for people who have experienced *transient ischemic attacks* (TIAs)—very small vascular blockages that clear without any residual problems, but this issue is presently being investigated.

Coumadin and warfarin are also effective in preventing the development of venous thrombosis after hip and knee surgery, as well as major gynecologic surgery, usually maintaining the INR in the 2.0 to 3.0 range.

Genetic predisposition to clot formation can be an issue for some people. Given the complexity of the coagulation cascade, it is not surprising that—as for almost any medical condition—

some people are predisposed to develop clots more easily than normal. Most people do not become aware of this until they experience a clotting problem, at which time it is often found that close relatives have had the same experience. Depending on the situation, these individuals may need to take an oral anticoagulant on a long-term basis, or they may only need the same three to six months of treatment after a clotting episode as is commonly used.

Section II

Successful Anticoagulation Management

THIS SECTION is the core of *The Coumadin® (Warfarin) Help Book*. Here's where you'll find detailed information about the daily management of your medication. These chapters discuss how these medications should be taken, how they should be monitored, and their side effects.

Because the major causes of problems with maintaining your INR level relate to changes in diet and medication, detailed information is provided about these issues. A chapter on how other medical conditions can affect the management of your anticoagulant—ranging from short-term issues such as the flu, to longer-term medical issues—provides guidelines and suggestions that will help you successfully navigate these tricky waters.

4

How Should I Take Coumadin or Warfarin?

INITIATING ANTICOAGULATION THERAPY

When you are first treated with Coumadin® or warfarin, it takes approximately five days for the medication to reach its full therapeutic effect, as measured by the INR being in the therapeutic range, most commonly 2.0 to 3.0. Unlike aspirin for a headache or an antibiotic for an infection, this long-acting anticoagulant must achieve a "steady state" level in the blood, which means its absorption and rate of degradation are in balance. The same is true for most drugs that affect a basic metabolic process in the body, such as hormones. This class of drugs has what is termed a "long half-life." To maintain therapeutic levels, the drug is first slowly increased to the desired level, after which daily additional doses are used to maintain that level.

Additionally, it is not safe to give what are termed "loading doses" of an oral long-acting anticoagulant—defined as 10 mg or more per day—in order to achieve the therapeutic level more rapidly. This can increase the risk of bleeding episodes early in therapy by eliminating or severely reducing the production of one of the essential factors in the body's own clotting system (Factor VII). It also increases the risk of other serious side effects.

For this reason, the initial dose of Coumadin or warfarin that you will usually be given is approximately the amount that is expected to be the *chronic maintenance dose* that you will take. For most people, the average maintenance dose is 4 to 6 mg per day. Dosages are inversely related to age, with lower doses usually given to older individuals. This is because overall metabolism slows with age, and the drug is removed from the body more slowly.

If you need anticoagulation but have not experienced a medical condition as a result of clotting—as would be the case, for example, in people with stable chronic atrial fibrillation (AF)—you will probably be started on an oral anticoagulant as an outpatient, without also requiring heparin (a fast-acting anticoagulant).

If you have experienced a clotting-related issue, such as a stroke, heart attack, or pulmonary embolism, initial therapy is most often a combination of two anticoagulants: fast-acting heparin and slower-acting Coumadin or warfarin. This means that you will be immediately protected against another clotting event. First, heparin is given by injection or intravenously, and then Coumadin or warfarin therapy is begun. The INR will be measured daily, or even more frequently, until it is in the desired range. As the INR rises to the therapeutic level, the amount of heparin will be gradually decreased and then stopped.

Based on recent research, it may be possible in the relatively near future to use genetic testing to identify individuals who may be more or less sensitive than average to Coumadin or warfarin. Such testing is based on measuring one of the enzymes involved in the coagulation cascade. Theoretically, it would allow physicians to determine those individuals who might benefit from a lower- or higher-than-usual initial dose, allowing them to achieve an optimal dosage earlier. However, it is not yet clear how useful such testing might be, or whether it has the potential to alter clinical practice.

Maintaining Your Correct Level of Anticoagulant Medication

Because it is so important to maintain your blood levels of Coumadin or warfarin within a very narrow range in your blood—usually an INR of 2.0 to 3.0—it is important to *take your medication exactly as prescribed.* If you have just started on anticoagulant therapy, you might be finding it difficult to keep your INR in the right range, and you might require frequent monitoring. Depending on the condition for which you are taking an oral anticoagulant, you might gradually be able to go for monitoring at longer intervals as you become more familiar with the foods and drugs that can affect keeping your level steady. While occasional changes might be necessary to your dose, with time, you will be able to avoid any major fluctuations in level.

Conversely, many people benefit from more frequent monitoring, either at home or in a doctor's office or clinic—especially people who are older, those who have medical conditions other than the one for which they are taking an oral anticoagulant, and those who are taking multiple medications. Your physician or nurse will work with you to determine the best option for your specific needs.

Keeping your levels steady and within the therapeutically effective range—remember, too low and the drug is ineffective; too high and you increase your risk of bleeding—will be much easier if you follow a few simple guidelines:

▶ Take your medication exactly as it was prescribed and at the dose prescribed.

▶ Store it at room temperature and away from moisture and heat.

▶ Do not switch between Coumadin and a generic medication without talking to your doctor or pharmacist. If you are taking generic warfarin, talk to your pharmacist about her policy on ordering generics from the same source. As discussed in more detail in Chapter 4, brand-name Coumadin and generics contain the same amount of active ingredient, but different formulations can have slightly different absorption properties, which can affect your blood levels of the active medication and thus the INR.

▶ To be sure your blood levels remain within the therapeutic range, do not miss any scheduled visits to your health care provider for blood testing. Most often, this takes only a few minutes, and it often can be done with a finger stick rather than a blood draw. If you are on home monitoring, be sure you test your levels regularly, and contact your health care provider if they are out of range. Remember, the monitor will only help if you use it!

▶ Take your medication at the same time every day. What works for me is to use a weekly pill holder with each day marked, keep it next to my toothbrush, and take the medication when I brush my teeth at night. With a bit of experimentation, you will find a system that works for *you*.

▶ Although Coumadin or warfarin can be taken with or without food, you will probably get the best result taking your medication on an empty stomach, because taking it with meals can lead to more variable amounts of the drug being absorbed, depending on what you eat.

▶ If you miss a dose, check with your physician or nurse. They will advise you if it is safe to take the dose late, or whether you should skip it or modify your schedule to maintain your levels in the desired range. *Never double up on your dose the next day, and don't change the dose on your own to make up for the missed dose.*

▶ Your body's response to Coumadin or warfarin can be affected by changes in your diet, changes in your environment, other medicines, or herbal products such as nutritional supplements, as well as your overall health. Contact your physician or nurse if you experience major changes, such as having the flu or if you need to take a new medication. Be careful not to become overheated in hot weather, and be sure to keep well hydrated, as a loss of fluid can alter your blood levels of medication.

▶ Seek medical attention if you think you have taken too much medication; especially, call your health care provider if you have accidentally taken a double dose.

▶ Be sure to get your prescription refilled well before you run out; if you do run out, and you normally get your prescriptions filled by mail, call your provider to have an emergency supply prescribed through a local pharmacy.

▶ If you need any type of surgery, or a procedure such as a colonoscopy that might involve a risk of bleeding, you might need to temporarily stop taking your medication. Be sure that any new physician or surgeon knows that you are using this medication.

▶ Carry an ID card such as MedicAlert® (http://www.med-icalert.org) or wear a medical alert bracelet stating that you are taking Coumadin or warfarin. In case of an emergency, any medical care provider who treats you will know that you are taking this medication and can take appropriate steps to prevent excessive bleeding—most likely by injecting synthetic vitamin K (Mephyton®), which is available only by prescription.

WHO SHOULD *NOT* TAKE COUMADIN OR WARFARIN?

Some medical conditions present problems and risks that outweigh the benefits of an oral anticoagulant. Most of them involve an existing risk of bleeding that might be increased by any drug that reduces clotting, making the danger of hemorrhage greater than the potential benefits of treatment.

Unless your doctor believes that the benefits outweigh the risks, he will generally not prescribe the drug if you have any of the following conditions:

▶ A tendency to hemorrhage due an abnormal blood condition, a stomach ulcer, or abnormal bleeding from the intestines, respiratory tract, or the genital or urinary system

▶ Bleeding of brain blood vessels, or a history of transient ischemic attacks (TIAs) that indicates a risk for hemorrhagic stroke—the type of stroke caused by blood vessel damage and leakage—in contrast to the ischemic type of stroke caused by a clot

▶ An aneurysm (a balloon-like swelling of a blood vessel associated with thinning of the vessel wall) in the brain, heart, or elsewhere in the vascular system

▶ A variety of heart and vascular system conditions, including inflammation due to bacterial infection of the membrane that lines the inside of the heart, inflammation of the membranes that surround the heart, an escape of fluid from the heart, and *malignant hypertension*—extremely elevated blood pressure that damages the inner linings of blood vessels, as well as the heart, spleen, kidneys, and brain

▶ A stomach ulcer or bleeding in the stomach (you might be able to take anticoagulant medication when and if these conditions have been corrected)

▶ Recent or contemplated surgery, or a medical procedure that can be associated with uncontrollable bleeding; if you are already taking Coumadin or warfarin and require such a procedure, you will be taken off the drug temporarily (see Chapter 9)

▶ An allergy to any of the drug's ingredients

▶ An inability to follow close directions and routinely keep doctor and lab appointments

▶ Alcoholism; the breakdown of alcohol by the body involves the same systems as warfarin, and its use can lead to dangerously high levels of the drug as well as to liver damage that can make it impossible to metabolize an anticoagulant normally.

Pregnancy

Pregnancy and breast-feeding present special issues for women taking anticoagulants. If you are a woman of childbearing age, you should use an effective form of birth control while you are taking an anticoagulant, discuss whether it is safe for you to become pregnant should you desire a child, and tell your doctor if you become pregnant during treatment. For more detail on this, see page 68.

COUMADIN OR GENERIC WARFARIN—WHICH SHOULD I USE?

As we have all seen in the past decade or so, there is usually a difference in the amount of our medical insurance co-pays—sometimes significant—between taking a brand-name drug and a generic product. What *really* is the difference?

The company that does the research and develops a brand-name drug through all of the stages that lead to approval by the U.S. Food and Drug Administration (FDA) has an exclusive right to sell the drug when it is first made available. This helps to compensate the company for the time and expense incurred in developing the drug—which can run to many millions of dollars and take six or seven years. After this period has expired, other companies can apply to the FDA for a license to produce the medication. These companies are able to sell the drug at a lower cost because they do not need to repeat the expensive animal and clinical research done by the original manufacturer to establish the drug's safety and effectiveness.

The basic issue when considering whether to take a brand-name or generic product is that the two versions should provide the same amount of active substance. This is normally the case; the generic product must meet quality-control specifications and tablet content uniformity standards—meaning a 2.5 mg tablet of either brand-name or generic will indeed contain 2.5 mg.

A potential problem arises when the issue of *bioequivalence* is considered, which means that the rate and extent of a generic drug's absorption in the body must be similar to those of the original brand-name drug. Differences in bioequivalence are caused by the exact formulation of the tablets, which can produce very slight differences in the way it is absorbed from the gut or metabolized by the body. In general, a generic drug will be maintained within a 90 percent "confidence interval," but even a 10 percent difference can cause a problem in the case of some drugs, such as Coumadin or warfarin, that have a narrow range of efficacy.

For many drugs, especially those taken for a short period of time to deal with a temporary problem, there is no noticeable difference between the brand-name or generic version. This is the case, for example, with many antibiotics or pain medications. For drugs that must be taken over a long period of time, it is important that the level of the drug in the body be maintained at a consistent level in order to obtain the desired effect in a consistent manner. Medicines that fall into this category include those taken for chronic conditions, such as high blood pressure, diabetes, or thyroid deficiency.

The same is true for the anticoagulant medication Coumadin and its generic version warfarin. As is the case with medications used for some other conditions, these drugs have what is referred to as a "narrow therapeutic index (or window)." This means that the desired effect of the drug—in this case to prevent excessive clotting without causing dangerous bleeding—is seen only when it is maintained within a narrow range. In the case of Coumadin and warfarin, it is very important to maintain the INR within a narrow range, 2.0 to 3.0 in most cases.

Switching a person whose INR is stable on Coumadin to generic warfarin—or the reverse—could potentially increase or decrease the clotting level, which could lead to bleeding if the INR increases or to clot formation if it decreases. This does *not* mean that you cannot successfully manage your clotting levels on a generic; it *does* mean that you should not switch from brand-name Coumadin to a generic without careful monitoring during the transition.

The same is true for switching between different sources of the generic medication. Since there are presently eleven manufacturers of warfarin in the United States, and given the definition of bioequivalence from 80 to 120 percent of Coumadin, switching manufacturers poses at least a theoretical problem. In reality, this wide range is usually much narrower, but still of concern.

Experienced pharmacists understand this issue and dispense accordingly. For any drug with a narrow window of efficacy, my own pharmacist makes sure that prescriptions are always filled with the same brand of generic. He follows guidelines that recommend pharmacists consider their ability to maintain an adequate supply of whichever manufacturer's drug is dispensed, in order to maintain the consistency of the patient's drug therapy. If possible, be sure that you always use the same pharmacy, and check with your pharmacist to make sure that this careful practice is followed.

If, like me, you usually get the prescriptions you use on a long-term basis from one of the large pharmacies associated with insurance companies, check their policy on this practice as well. When I checked with the company that provides my medications, one of the largest in the United States, I was told that they purchase *all* drugs, including those with a narrow window of efficacy, from whichever company charges the least at the time the order is placed or for a defined contract period. Bottom line: Be sure your monitoring is done frequently enough to allow any changes in INR caused by a switch of manufacturer to be detected as soon as possible.

Be sure your monitoring is done frequently enough to allow any changes in INR caused by a switch of manufacturer to be detected as soon as possible.

Once you are stable on either the brand-name drug or a generic, you should have little difficulty keeping your INR in the appropriate range, provided that you follow your physician's instructions and the dietary and drug guidelines given elsewhere in this book.

5

Monitoring: Maintaining Your Clotting Rate in the Desired Range

B ECAUSE IT IS SO IMPORTANT to maintain the time in which your blood clots in the narrow range called a *therapeutic window,* you will need frequent blood tests when you first begin taking Coumadin® or warfarin. If your blood levels remain stable, this interval can be lengthened to once every four to six weeks, although some people need to continue with more frequent testing. Only your physician knows what is right for you. It is not a good idea to go for any length of time without testing, because a wide range of factors, including changes in diet and illness, can affect blood levels.

Also, measuring your INR regularly gives you a "report card" on how well you are managing your medication. The very fact that—unlike most drugs—you get regular feedback means that what physicians call "compliance" is higher with oral anticoagulants than with many other drugs. It is not easy to slack off taking your medications as prescribed when you know the next test is coming up!

As discussed earlier, the *International Normalized Ratio*, or INR, measures clotting time in a standardized way that takes into account differences in age, gender, and testing method. Most people need to keep their INR in the 2.0 to 3.0 range; others have a higher-than-normal risk of clot formation and need to maintain a slightly higher INR, in the 2.5 to 3.5 range. This is an increase from the INR of approximately 1.0 in people who are not taking an oral anticoagulant.

Measuring your INR regularly gives you a "report card" on how well you are managing your medication.

As discussed earlier, since Coumadin and generic warfarin differ slightly in the way they are absorbed and metabolized by the body, your INR levels will need to be measured more often if you switch from Coumadin to generic warfarin, or the reverse. If a specific brand of generic warfarin is started and then used exclusively, it is likely to be as safe as Coumadin, but pharmacies sometimes change the source of their generic product based on price. For this reason, don't switch pharmacists without good reason once you are stabilized on your medication.

IS HOME MONITORING RIGHT FOR ME?

Home monitoring might be a viable option, depending on your particular situation. If it is difficult for you to make regular trips to have testing done, or you live in a rural area, home monitoring can increase your ability to control your medication and maintain a stable INR. People who are well-controlled with a stable INR, and who can be relied on to monitor themselves, are also good candidates for home monitoring (I meet these criteria, and my Coumadin nurse has recommended home monitoring).

For some people, weekly monitoring increases their chances of remaining within the desired INR range, as compared with less frequent testing. This is especially true for older individuals, people who are taking multiple medications, and people with serious medical conditions in addition to the one for which they are taking an oral anticoagulant.

When your dosage needs to be adjusted, too frequent testing can provide incorrect information. It takes a certain amount of time for the INR to stabilize after a change in dosage levels is made, and the desired level might not have been achieved by the time the next test is done. In general, no additional changes in dosage should be made until the last one has had time to take effect, generally a minimum of seven days.

For some people, weekly monitoring increases their chances of remaining within the desired range.

If your physician feels that weekly monitoring is appropriate for you, it can be easily done at home, and you should discuss this option with her. The test can be easily performed either by the person needing testing or by a family member or friend. Monitors and testing strips are both prescription items, and they can only be obtained with your physician's support. People who test their INR at home are trained to do so by their physician or nurse, or by the company providing the monitor (see Resources).

Remember that home INR testing *complements*—it does not replace—your ongoing relationship with the physician who manages your overall health, as well as the condition for which you are taking an anticoagulant! Your regular physician visits are critical to your optimal health.

Medicare and many private health insurers cover home INR testing, but not necessarily for all conditions and sometimes only for a specific brand of monitor. Some insurance companies follow the guidelines for home monitoring set by Medicare. In March 2008, Medicare expanded its coverage of home monitoring to include people with mechanical heart valves, atrial fibrillation (AF), and venous thromboembolism. To qualify for home testing via Medicare, you will need to have taken anticoagulation medication for at least three months, attend an educational program on anticoagulation management, demonstrate the correct use of the device, continue to use it correctly, and use it no more frequently than once a week.

FUTURE ALTERNATIVES TO COUMADIN AND WARFARIN?

Several new oral anticoagulant drugs in the testing stage may be easier to manage than Coumadin or warfarin. One, Apixaban®, is currently being tested for the prevention of venous thromboembolism. It is hoped that this drug, as well as others now in various stages of development, might be easier to manage and have fewer side effects.

Such drugs would be expected to be many times more expensive than Coumadin or warfarin. However, should one or more of them prove to be as effective, this strong negative will have to be weighed against the full costs of managing their use. This includes the need for frequent testing and the costs of managing what medical people refer to—somewhat inadequately—as "adverse events" associated with not keeping the INR in the appropriate range.

6

Side Effects of Oral Anticoagulant Therapy

A NUMBER OF SIDE EFFECTS—mostly easily manageable but sometimes serious—can result from Coumadin® or warfarin therapy. Some side effects are more common early in treatment, when the optimal level has not yet been achieved; others tend to occur only after a prolonged period on therapy.

One caution that applies to anyone with a chronic medical issue: A natural tendency exists to blame any medical symptom on a condition for which you are being actively treated, or on a medication that you take regularly, especially if it is difficult to manage. In reality, everyone on a medication such as an anticoagulant can develop any of the many illnesses to which we are all subject. For example, bleeding when the INR is under 3 is often associated with an ulcer or other lesion in the GI tract or kidney, not as a direct result of oral anticoagulant therapy.

Do *not* assume that any new medical problems are the result of your anticoagulant medication or the medical problem for which it was prescribed. This means you need to get regular medical checkups and tests, from Pap smears and prostate exams to colonoscopies. Routine preventive medical care is discussed in more detail in Chapter 10, which includes a summary of recommendations for the routine examinations that everyone should have.

Do not assume that any new medical problems are the result of your anticoagulant medication or the medical problem for which it was prescribed.

With this in mind, here are some of the side effects (both common and rare) that can result from anticoagulant therapy. We also refer you to the product information that comes with your medication, or you can download it from the Internet at http://www.coumadin.com.

BLEEDING

The major complication associated with Coumadin and warfarin is bleeding due to excessive anticoagulation. For most conditions for which these drugs are prescribed, "excessive" means an INR of greater than 3.0. That's why it is so very important to have your INR measured regularly and to follow dietary and drug management guidelines. Excessive bleeding, or *hemorrhage*, can occur from any area of the body. Contact your physician if you experience a fall or accident—even if you don't have any obvious injury—or have any signs of bleeding or bruising. These signs might include:

▶ Blood in the stool or black tarry stool
▶ Red or dark brown urine
▶ Bleeding of the gums when you brush your teeth
▶ Nosebleeds
▶ Coughing up blood

▸ Decreased urine production
▸ Bleeding when you cut yourself that doesn't stop or takes an unusually long time to stop
▸ Bruising under the skin
▸ Purple discoloration of the toes or fingers
▸ A heavy or prolonged menstrual period
▸ Unusual bleeding, bruising, swelling, pain, or discomfort anywhere on your body

Although any of these symptoms could be related to problems other than a high INR, they all warrant medical attention.

Also, be sure to contact your physician or nurse after a fall to be evaluated for possible internal injury. I had a major fall while hiking Mayan ruins in Honduras, far away from any medical treatment; fortunately, no subsequent problem occurred, but it was most definitely *not* ideal!

> *Contact your physician or nurse after a fall to be evaluated for possible internal injury*

Bleeding is more likely to occur in people who need to take higher doses of anticoagulant and need to maintain an INR over 3.0.

There are some simple things you can do to reduce bleeding:

▸ Use a softer toothbrush and waxed rather than unwaxed floss if you have problems with bleeding gums.
▸ Shave with an electric razor rather than a blade.
▸ Avoid potentially harmful activities such as contact sports, or sports such as skiing that have the potential for serious injury.
▸ Be especially careful when handling tools of any sort, including kitchen knives.

▶ Be careful working around the house; for example, people on anticoagulant therapy have experienced falls off roofs and ladders and experienced serious bleeding as a result.

▶ Prevent falls in your home by using nonskid rugs, moving all electrical cords so they will not cause you to trip, removing clutter from stairways and other areas, and using night lights to illuminate hallways and bathrooms.

RISKS OF BLEEDING IN OLDER INDIVIDUALS

Bleeding is more likely during anticoagulation treatment for people over 65, and it is more likely to occur during the first few weeks of treatment. A physician will need to consider whether the risk of anticoagulation outweighs the potential benefit of therapy in an elderly person, especially if that person has any cognitive impairment and might not take his medication properly, thus running the risk of a bleeding episode. As with everyone on this therapy, the best results are obtained by careful monitoring and maintaining an INR between 2.0 and 3.0. Home monitoring at frequent intervals by a family member or other caregiver can be helpful in avoiding problems.

Bleeding is more likely during anticoagulation treatment for people over 65, and it is more likely to occur during the first few weeks of treatment.

IF YOUR INR IS SIGNIFICANTLY ELEVATED

If your INR level is above 3 (or 3.5, if that is your desired range) but less than 6, you will most probably be asked to simply cut back on your dosage and have your INR tested frequently until you are stabilized in the normal range. Higher levels are usually treated with *prothrombin complex concentrate* (PCC) and/or intravenously administered vitamin K (Mephyton®), which will immediately stimulate the clotting system. This procedure is done most commonly in the emergency room, but, in some cases, might require a brief hospital stay to make sure that no major bleeding event occurs while the level is high. Vitamin K should *never* be self-administered in case of injury or for any excessive bleeding.

If you are given a prescription for Mephyton, be sure you stay in close contact with the prescribing physician or nurse until your INR has returned to the normal range. During this period, you should take extra safety precautions to prevent bumps, bruises, cuts, and falls.

It is important to determine the cause of your significantly increased INR, so that you can prevent the problem from recurring. A careful review of your diet and medications is in order.

WHAT IF MY INR IS TOO LOW?

You are probably taking Coumadin or warfarin because you have already experienced a stroke, heart attack, PE, or other cardiovascular problem, and you need to prevent another. Or, you are taking anticoagulants to prevent any of these "adverse events" from occurring in the first place because you have a predisposing condition, such as an arrhythmia. To do this, you must keep your INR above 2.0. If it drops below this level, you will not have adequate protection against the development of blood clots.

If your INR tests below 2.0, your dosage probably will be increased by an amount that your health care provider believes will quickly restore your clotting ability to the desired level, then reduced back to the level expected to maintain the INR in this range. It is important that you have your INR checked frequently until everyone is sure that you are on the right dose and your level is being maintained in the correct range.

OTHER COMPLICATIONS OF ANTICOAGULATION THERAPY

Anticoagulant therapy can have other effects. In addition to any signs of bleeding, call your doctor if you experience any of the following:

- ▶ A skin rash or irritation
- ▶ An unusual fever
- ▶ Persistent nausea or gastrointestinal upset
- ▶ Dizziness, headache, or weakness
- ▶ Pain in your joints or back
- ▶ An allergic reaction (difficulty breathing; closing of the throat; swelling of the lips, tongue, or face; or hives)
- ▶ Excessive gas or bloating
- ▶ Decreased appetite or weight

Again, any of these symptoms might be unrelated to your medication, but all warrant being checked by your physician.

Weight Gain

A review of chat rooms and other Internet sites shows that weight gain is commonly reported as a side effect of Coumadin or warfarin therapy. However, the weight gain might be due to limitations on activity because of the underlying problem for which anticoagulant therapy is needed or for many other reasons. If you have recently gained weight, discuss it with your primary care provider, who might do a series of tests to establish the cause of your weight gain and/or refer you to a nutritionist.

Hair Loss

Hair loss appears to be a common side effect of anticoagulant therapy. This is rarely severe, and complete hair loss doesn't usually occur, but it can be distressing. I've experienced some hair loss, and am delighted that recently it seems to have regrown—this appears to be common with time. Hair loss due to Coumadin or warfarin therapy almost always reverses when the therapy is stopped—but, of course, this is *not* a good reason to stop therapy!

Some people experience hair loss, not because of the drug, but as the result of a stroke or other major clotting episode such as a pulmonary embolism. Since hair loss might not occur until some time afterwards, people tend to assume that the anticoagulant therapy was responsible. This type of hair loss also tends to reverse over time.

OSTEOPOROSIS

There appears to be an increased risk of osteoporosis in older men and women taking an oral anticoagulant, with a 25 percent increase in the frequency of hip fractures seen in people whose average age is 80. Vitamin K plays an essential role in maintaining healthy bone tissue, and it helps prevent osteoporosis. These are both good reasons to continue enjoying those vitamin K–containing leafy greens and vegetables. You can adjust your dosage of anticoagulant to accommodate them—always remembering to be consistent—but you can't easily undo the effects of osteoporosis!

RARE BUT SERIOUS SIDE EFFECTS

Necrosis (an area of dying tissue) is a rare complication of anti-coagulant therapy. It occurs in people who have a deficiency of one of the proteins involved in the clotting cascade, and might be accompanied by dark red or black lesions on the skin. Necrosis is most likely to occur during the first several days of anticoagulant therapy, especially if a high dose is given. This should not occur if the initial dose is low and increased gradually, or as a combination of heparin and low doses of Coumadin or warfarin. The dose of oral anticoagulant is gradually increased and that of heparin decreased, until the INR is in the right range

Another rare complication that can occur early during anticoagulant treatment (usually within three to eight weeks) is *purple toe syndrome.* This condition is thought to result from small deposits of cholesterol breaking loose and flowing into the blood vessels in the skin of the feet, which causes a bluish purple color and can be painful. It is typically thought to affect the big toe, but it can affect other parts of the feet as well, including the bottom of the foot (plantar surface). If this condition occurs, anticoagulant therapy might need to be discontinued, at least temporarily.

OTHER SIDE EFFECTS

Side effects other than those discussed here can also occur. Talk to your doctor about any problem that seems unusual or that is especially bothersome.

7

Dietary Considerations with Oral Anticoagulant Therapy

A S WE DISCUSSED in Chapter 1, the vitamin K in your diet affects the blood clotting process. If you eat a lot of foods that are high in vitamin K, the effect of your anticoagulant will be reduced, and your INR might drop below the therapeutic range. Conversely, reducing foods that contain vitamin K intake can increase the anticoagulant's effect, raising your INR levels and increasing the possibility of a bleeding episode.

In general, leafy green vegetables, some legumes, and some vegetable oils contain high amounts of vitamin K. Foods that are low in vitamin K include roots, bulbs, tubers, grains, the fleshy part of fruits, fruit juices, and other beverages.

Here is a guideline, by food group, to vitamin K content:

▶ Vegetables are the group of foods you need to be most concerned about. As a general "rule of thumb," the greener the vegetable, the more likely it is to contain substantial amounts of vitamin K. This includes lettuce and other "leafy greens" such as kale, broccoli, Brussels sprouts, and cabbage. Vegetables such as corn or carrots are relatively low in vitamin K content, and some vegetables have a medium level.

▶ Some oils, such as canola oil, are high in vitamin K; safflower and corn oil are low in vitamin K.

▶ Essentially all grain products, fruits, and dairy products are low in vitamin K; you can eat them in normal amounts without concern.

▶ Most meats are low in vitamin K, with the exception of liver (where all those clotting factors are made).

Two good Internet sources with more detailed information about the vitamin K content of a variety of foods are http://www.drgourmet.com/askdrgourmet/warfarin/index.shtml and http://www.ptinr.com/data/pages/vkregistry.aspx.

You might ask whether it would be easier to avoid vitamin K, rather than worrying about eating the same amount every day. However, *all* vitamins are necessary for life, and limiting your intake of any of them is most definitely not a good idea! Leafy green vegetables provide important nutrients needed in your diet, and you should *not* avoid them because of concern that they will alter your INR.

Leafy green vegetables provide important nutrients needed in your diet, and you should not avoid them because of concern that they will alter your INR.

The key to managing your diet is just that—to *manage* it. The most important issue while taking Coumadin® or warfarin is to maintain a healthy and *consistent* diet, and to keep the amount of vitamin K in your diet reasonably constant from day to day. For example, I make sure to have one serving of a leafy green, such as a salad, broccoli, or Brussels sprouts every day, and my Coumadin dose reflects this—just as it reflects the medications I take on a daily basis.

If you are having difficulty keeping your INR constant, try keeping a food diary, which over a period of several weeks will show either that you are eating vitamin K–containing foods on an irregular basis, or that you have been eating foods containing vitamin K without realizing it. A convenient food diary form can be downloaded from www.ptinr.com.

In general, once your INR is stable, you should not make any major changes to your diet without consulting your physician or nurse. You should also tell your health care provider if an illness causes your diet to change. Also, contact your provider if you have an illness such as the flu, which can disrupt your normal fluid balance and also affect the ability of the bacteria in your gut to synthesize vitamin K.

Remember, the amount of vitamin K that you take in each day adds up. If you eat a lot of foods that contain a medium amount of vitamin K in a single day, your vitamin K intake will be high that day.

Most importantly, *relax!* Slight variations won't have a major effect over time, as long as you always return to those key principles of consistency and moderation.

8

How Do Drugs and Supplements
Affect Coumadin or Warfarin Levels?

M ANY FACTORS CAN AFFECT the way your body responds to anticoagulant therapy. Managing your dose of Coumadin® and warfarin is complicated by the fact that they interact with many commonly used medications. Interactions with a wide range of drugs is second only to the vitamin K content of your diet in terms of their potential to cause problems in maintaining your INR in the desired range, and your medications will need to be monitored closely.

As noted previously, drugs that you take every day for disorders such as high blood pressure and thyroid abnormalities, and diseases such as diabetes, are less likely to cause problems than those that you need to take on a short-term basis, such as antibiotics for an infection. This is because the medications you take consistently can be easily compensated for in your daily dose of Coumadin or warfarin. Your initial therapy regimen, in which your base dosage is determined, will take these into account. A short-term need will probably mean more frequent

INR level measurements during the course of therapy, with the dosage modified as needed.

Some drug interactions are the result of a drug's being degraded in the liver by the same enzymes that metabolize Coumadin or warfarin. These are called the *cytochrome P450 enzymes*. When these enzymes are actively involved in metabolizing other drugs, they are less able to metabolize the anticoagulant—essentially they "compete" for the enzymes' attention. By slowing degradation of the anticoagulant drug, these interactions result in an increase in the amount of anticoagulant medication in the body, and thus slow the rate of clotting and increase the INR—sometimes into the range in which the risk of a bleeding episode is seriously increased.

Drug–drug interactions with oral anticoagulants are classified as either *pharmacokinetic* or *pharmacodynamic*. Pharmacokinetic interactions can involve changes in the way a drug is absorbed, bound to proteins, or metabolized by the liver. Pharmacodynamic interactions alter the risk of bleeding or clotting by altering platelet aggregation or vitamin K metabolism.

COMMONLY USED DRUGS THAT CAN ALTER THE EFFECTS OF ORAL ANTICOAGULANTS ON THE INR

Most commonly used drugs that can affect the INR do so through their effect on liver enzymes and also on the level of bacteria in the gut. Others decrease clotting because they inhibit platelet function. A number of websites have detailed information about potential interactions with drugs, including http://www.coumadin.com and http://www.rxlist.com/cgi/

generic/warfarin_ad.htm. The following summarizes some of the main drug types that can affect the INR.

Nonsteroidal Anti-inflammatory Drugs

The group of drugs called *nonsteroidal anti-inflammatory drugs* (NSAIDs) is commonly prescribed for inflammation due to arthritis and other conditions. These drugs affect platelet function and significantly increase the risk of gastrointestinal bleeding in people on anticoagulant therapy. This combination is at the top of the list of the ten most dangerous drug interactions, and it is partially responsible for the Black-Box Warning associated with Coumadin and warfarin. These drugs include aspirin, ibuprofen (Motrin®), naproxen (Aleve®, Naprosyn®), and many others. Of these, aspirin is the most important because of its widespread use and prolonged effect.

It is important to realize that impaired platelet function is not reflected in the INR, and the increased risk of bleeding will not likely be detected with normal monitoring. This makes it especially important that you work with your health care provider to achieve relief of symptoms safely.

Any drug prescribed to reduce inflammation, pain, and fever falls into this category, so you should check with your doctor before taking them. Acetaminophen (Tylenol®) has less of an interaction than other drugs in this group, so it is often suggested as the first choice for pain. However, be aware that Tylenol can be a dangerous and even fatal drug when taken in excess over a prolonged period of time, which can easily occur if it is combined with other acetaminophen-containing medications such as cold preparations. Your physician might prescribe a mild narcotic or other medication as an alternative for managing pain.

Cox-2 Inhibitors

Cox-2–specific inhibitors such as Celebrex® are considered NSAIDs, but they have only a minimal effect on platelet function and can reduce the incidence of gastrointestinal bleeding in people taking anticoagulants. However, Celebrex has been associated with increases in INR and bleeding events. More frequent INR testing is recommended to make sure that any interactions are caught early, and to avoid or greatly minimize the potential for a bleeding event. Individuals needing a Cox-2 medication are often stabilized on a lower dose of anticoagulant medication.

Sulfa Drugs and Antibiotics

One of the most important groups of drugs that can affect clotting includes many commonly used sulfa drugs and antibiotics. These can greatly increase the effect of your anticoagulant medication by reducing the metabolism of Coumadin and warfarin. They have the same effect as decreasing vitamin K in the diet—they increase the effect of anticoagulants as reflected by an increase in the INR, and thus they increase the potential of a bleeding episode. Whenever you are prescribed a drug to treat an infection of any kind, be sure the physician prescribing it knows that you are taking an oral anticoagulant, and contact your Coumadin/warfarin provider to discuss whether the dosage should be modified, and whether more frequent INR testing would be appropriate.

This group of drugs includes (but is not limited to) Bactrim®, Biaxin®, Cipro®, erythromycin (and other antibiotics whose name ends in "mycin"), the broad-spectrum penicillins, and the tetracy-clines. In addition to their effect on anticoagulant metabolism, some antibi-otics also reduce the number of bacteria found in the bowel, which make signifi-cant quantities of vitamin K2. As already noted, sulfa drugs and a wide variety of commonly used antibi-otics can require a reduction in your anticoagulant dose by as much as 50 percent. These drugs also cause among the most seri-ous drug interactions and are part of the reason for the Black-Box Warning that comes with Coumadin and warfarin prescriptions.

Whenever you are prescribed a drug to treat an infection of any kind, be sure the physician prescribing it knows that you are taking an oral anticoagulant.

Other Drugs

Other classes of drug known to interact with oral anticoagu-lants include antiepileptic medications, hormones such as Synthroid® or generic levothyroxine, and some antidepres-sants. If taken on a daily basis, these medications can be easily adjusted for over time.

A very few drugs can increase the rate of elimination of Coumadin and warfarin, causing the INR to decrease and reducing the effectiveness of the anticoagulants. The main drugs that have been identified as having this effect are used to reduce cholesterol and other fatty substances in the blood; they include Cholestyramine® and Colestipol®.

The "bottom line" is to check with the health care provider responsible for your overall care before taking any new medication. She will consider potential drug interactions before prescribing any new medications, and will also carefully monitor medications prescribed by other physicians.

Colds and Flu Medications

As noted earlier, colds and flu can alter your overall metabolism and affect the way Coumadin or warfarin is handled in the body. This can increase bleeding time, as reflected by the INR. If possible, when you become ill with a cold or the flu, you should have an INR test when you are able.

Most cold and flu medications contain acetaminophen (Tylenol) and other drugs to ease symptoms. It is important not to take them excessively. Be especially careful of cough drops containing zinc, because zinc affects Coumadin and warfarin uptake from the digestive tract and can lower the INR.

Alcohol Abuse

As noted in Chapter 1, excessive alcohol use affects the metabolism of anticoagulant medications and can elevate the INR. It is important that you not use alcohol excessively while taking an oral anticoagulant.

Some physicians recommend not ingesting any alcohol while on anticoagulation therapy, while others—like my own

Coumadin/warfarin clinic—recommend that your alcohol intake should not exceed two drinks per day. Like medications and vitamin K–containing foods, consistency is the key. It is easier to adjust your dose of oral anticoagulant if you drink moderate amounts of alcohol regularly than if you use it irregularly, especially if you indulge in binge drinking.

People suffering from liver damage or alcoholism may need to be treated with heparin injections instead of an oral anticoagulant.

INTERACTIONS WITH HERBAL PREPARATIONS

The increased popularity of herbal remedies and *complementary and alternative medicine* (CAM) has created a growing number of concerns about their possible interactions with anticoagulants. Some herbal remedies appear to have the potential to enhance or decrease the action of anticoagulants, and some of them actually have anticoagulant properties. In either case, they have the potential to significantly alter the effects of your medication. For this reason, it is very important to discuss with your physician or nurse any herbal products that you use. At my Coumadin/warfarin clinic, starting, stopping, or changing herbal medications is one of the major reasons why INR fluctuations occur.

As noted elsewhere, you can take most medications, including herbal preparations, while on Coumadin or warfarin, but you need to take them *consistently*. It is of particular importance to remember that herbal preparations are not required to be standardized, and potency can vary significantly from one lot to another. Because of this, you should look for a brand that claims to be standardized, and use that brand consistently.

64 | THE COUMADIN® (WARFARIN) HELP BOOK

Most herbal medicines known to interfere with oral anti-coagulant therapy increase the INR and risk of bleeding. Some of them contain *coumarins*, which are similar to Coumadin or warfarin; some contain the aspirin-like substance *salicylate* and might also have antiplatelet properties; and some are true anti-coagulants. Do not use any of these products without first asking your doctor. Some of them affect platelet aggregation, and their effects will not be seen in the INR, which can make them of particular concern. These herbal agents include (but are not limited to):

▶ *Ginkgo* (or Ginkgo Biloba) is used to increase brain blood flow, prevent dementia, and improve memory.

▶ *Ginseng* is used to help with fatigue and weakness; in addition to its effect on the INR, it can increase blood pressure and heart rate.

▶ *Garlic* (as a supplement, not in the diet) is commonly used to help lower high cholesterol levels, high triglyc-erides, and high blood pressure.

▶ *Ginger* is commonly used to relieve nausea and poor digestion. It increases the risk of bleeding by inhibiting platelet aggregation.

A few herbal products, such as St. John's Wort (used to help with mild to moderate depression) and coenzyme Q10, have the opposite effect and decrease the INR.

9

Oral Anticoagulants and Other Medical Conditions

WHATEVER THE CONDITION for which Coumadin® or warfarin was prescribed, you are as likely as anyone else to develop a wide range of medical conditions and illnesses, many of which can affect the way anticoagulant medication affects your body.

For this reason, all of your physicians and other medical providers need to know that you are on anticoagulant therapy. Treatments given for any newly diagnosed condition can change the rate at which the drug is absorbed from the gut, metabolized by your liver, and excreted by your kidneys. If you are prescribed any new medication, you might need to have your blood levels checked more frequently until they are stabilized.

All of your physicians and other medical providers need to know that you are on anticoagulant therapy.

Any new medications that will be taken long-term, such as those for high blood pressure or a thyroid condition, will require one or two extra INR checks to determine whether changes in dosage are needed.

Medications taken short-term can alter your INR levels. Antibiotics are the most likely class of drugs to have a significant effect on your INR, because they are metabolized by liver enzymes, and because they deplete your gut of the bacteria that produce vitamin K2. Contact your physician or nurse to see if you should make any adjustments in your dosage while taking the new medication, and have your INR tested as they recommend during and after treatment.

Call your nurse or physician if you have a serious case of the flu, because the serious upset in both absorption from the gut and general loss of fluids can cause blood levels of oral anticoagulant to change dramatically

SURGERY AND NONINVASIVE MEDICAL PROCEDURES

If you require surgery for any reason, you will probably need to stop your anticoagulation therapy and switch to heparin for a few days before the surgery. I recently had a surgical repair on my shoulder and stopped taking Coumadin for a period of days. I also started taking what is termed "bridging" Lovenox®—an injectable form of heparin that clears from the system quickly, so that I would not bleed excessively during surgery. I stopped taking the Lovenox two days before the surgery, and then began taking my usual dose of Coumadin the day after, which slowly increased back to normal levels over about a week. This ensured that there was no excessive bleeding during or after the surgery. Individuals at high risk for clot formation may need to use Lovenox immediately after surgery to quickly restore their INR to the effective range.

It is important to be sure that the physician who manages the medical condition for which you take Coumadin or warfarin and the surgeon have communicated regarding your therapy and upcoming surgery.

The same applies to medical procedures that have the potential to cause bleeding, such as a colonoscopy. My own gastroenterologist is comfortable doing a colonoscopy without patients having to temporarily stop taking Coumadin or warfarin, and he would be able to remove a small polyp without concern. However, if he found a larger-sized polyp that needed to be removed, he would repeat the procedure to remove the polyp only after the patient had ceased taking oral anticoagulant medication for several days and used bridging Lovenox. Your physician might have a different view of the same situation, and in all cases, his advice should be followed.

MEDICAL EMERGENCIES

If you experience a fall or other injury, depending on its severity, you should go to the emergency room or visit your physician. Any uncontrolled bleeding, including blood in the urine or with a bowel movement, is also cause for an immediate checkup. An injury such as a deep bruise, even if it doesn't involve visible bleeding, is also reason to contact your physician or nurse.

If you need emergency surgery for any reason, be sure to tell the medical personnel involved that you take Coumadin or warfarin. They will administer vitamin K (Mephyton®) or prothrombin complex to reverse the effects of the drug so that surgery can be done safely and without excessive bleeding.

This is an excellent reason to wear a MedicAlert® bracelet or other piece of identification jewelry, and also to carry a card in your wallet indicating that you take anticoagulant medication. Should you ever be unconscious and in need of immediate care, emergency personnel are trained to take notice of this information, and they will be able to safely manage your care.

DENTAL CLEANING AND SURGERY

Routine teeth cleaning and procedures such as fillings generally do not warrant going off your anticoagulation therapy. Check with your physician and dentist about this. If you have a heart-related condition, your dentist will probably want you to take an antibiotic prior to cleaning.

Any dental procedure that involves the possibility of significant bleeding may require that you temporarily stop taking your anticoagulant medication. This would be the case, for example, with treatment for gum disease, implants, and extractions. You might need to temporarily stop taking your medication before cleaning, as well, if you have severe gum disease, with "spongy" gum tissue.

PREGNANCY

Coumadin or warfarin should not be taken by women who are or might become pregnant, because the drug passes through the placental barrier and can cause the fetus to have a fatal hemorrhage. Additionally, birth defects have been reported in children born to mothers who were treated with anticoagulants during pregnancy, and miscarriage and stillbirth can occur. Low birth weight and retarded growth after birth have also been reported. Contact the physician who manages your Coumadin or warfarin therapy immediately should you become pregnant.

Although anticoagulants do not pass into breast milk, you should consult your physician if you wish to breast-feed while taking an oral anticoagulant, because you and your baby might need additional monitoring.

This does not mean that it is impossible for you to have a child while on anticoagulant therapy. The most dangerous time for the development of birth defects is during the first trimester. If pregnancy is carefully planned, you might be able to stop taking your anticoagulant medication before becoming pregnant and during the first trimester. One of the nurses at my Coumadin/warfarin clinic is pregnant and used this strategy. At the time of this writing, she just had her baby and is again taking her medication, but she is not breast-feeding.

Everyone is different, and the condition for which you are taking anticoagulant medication might or might not make this a reasonable alternative. As always, *only your physician can help you to make this decision.*

Section III

General Health Concerns

IT IS IMPORTANT TO KEEP the need to manage your oral antico-agulant medication in perspective. It is only one part of managing your overall health, and it should not be such an overwhelming concern that you attribute any new medical issue to the medication or the condition for which you take it. You are just as subject to other problems as anyone else, so this section contains some general guidelines for managing your overall health.

This section also focuses on managing your anticoagulation therapy outside of the home. It's a wide world out there, and we encourage you to enjoy it!

10

Managing Your General Health

REMEMBER THAT, whatever the condition for which you are taking Coumadin® or warfarin, you are still subject to the same medical problems as everyone else. It is important that you watch your overall health—all those guidelines about healthy eating, getting exercise, not smoking, and getting regular checkups apply to YOU! Staying as healthy as possible will also help to prevent unnecessary problems with maintaining your anticoagulant therapy in the proper range.

What can you do to stay healthy and prevent disease? You can practice healthy behaviors, take medicines as prescribed, and get regular checkups and screening tests. When you go for your next checkup, talk to your primary care physician about what steps you can take to stay as healthy as possible.

Screening tests, such as a periodic colonoscopy, can find diseases early, when they are easier to treat. Some people need certain screening tests earlier, or more often, than others. Talk to your doctor about which of the tests in Table 10.1 are right for you, when you should have them, and how often. In addition to the guidelines that apply to everyone, we've provided separate information for men and women.

TABLE 10.1 HEALTH GUIDELINES FOR ALL ADULTS

▶ *Preventive Health Exam:* Age 19–40, every 5 years; 41–50 every 3 years; 51–59, every 2 years; 60+ every 1–2 years.

▶ *Blood Pressure and Pulse:* Yearly, if normal.

▶ *Tests for High Cholesterol:* As a generally guideline, you should have a fasting cholesterol (with HDL, LDL, and triglycerides) done every 5 years, and more frequently as your doctor recommends.

▶ *Routine Blood and Urine Tests:* These should be part of your regular physical exam, at an interval that your physician deems appropriate—generally once a year after 50. A test for thyroid function should be part of general testing, especially for women aged 40 and older.

▶ *Diabetes Tests:* Have a test to screen for diabetes if you have high blood pressure or high cholesterol. You should have a fasting blood sugar test done every 5 years, more frequently if your physician recommends it.

▶ *Colorectal Cancer Tests:* Begin regular screening for colorectal cancer starting at age 50. A stool smear test should be done yearly starting at age 50, and a colonoscopy should be done every 5 years on average.

▶ *Depression:* If you've felt "down," sad, or hopeless, and have had little interest or pleasure in doing things for 2 weeks straight, talk to your doctor about whether she will evaluate you for depression.

▶ *Sexually Transmitted Diseases:* Talk to your doctor to see whether you should be screened for sexually transmitted diseases, such as HIV.

▶ *Abdominal Aortic Aneurysm Screening:* If you have ever smoked, an ultrasound is recommended between the ages of 65–75 to check for aneurysms. (An *aneurysm* is a bulge in an artery wall; it is more common in men than women.)

▶ *Dental Cleaning and Exam:* At least yearly, and preferably every 6 months; check with your dentist for the frequency recommended for you.

▶ *Vision/Glaucoma:* Every 2–4 years for ages 40–65, and then yearly.

▶ *Hearing:* Every 5 years over age 50.

Medications That Can Help Prevent Disease

▶ *Aspirin:* Talk to your doctor about taking aspirin to help prevent heart disease if you are over 40, if you are younger than 40 and have high blood pressure, high cholesterol, or diabetes, or if you smoke.

▶ *Immunizations:* Stay up-to-date with your immunizations:

- Have a flu shot every year starting at age 50.
- Have a tetanus-diphtheria shot every 10 years.
- Have a pneumonia shot once at age 65 (you might need it earlier if you have certain health problems, such as pulmonary disease).
- Talk to your doctor to see whether you need hepatitis B shots.
- You might need supplemental immunizations, such as hepatitis A, in special circumstances, such as overseas travel to developing countries.

Special Concerns of Women

▶ *Mammograms:* Have a mammogram every 1–2 years starting at age 40, and yearly after age 50. If you have a family history of breast cancer, check with your physician about the appropriate age to begin getting mammograms and their recommended frequency. Be sure to do a manual breast exam monthly.

▶ *Pap Smears:* Have a Pap smear every 1–3 years, beginning at age 18, unless you have never been sexually active.

▶ *Osteoporosis Tests:* Have a bone density test every 5 years, starting at age 55, to screen for osteoporosis (a loss of calcium from the bones).

▶ *Chlamydia Tests:* Have a test for chlamydia if you are 25 or younger and sexually active. If you are older, talk to your doctor to see whether you should be tested.

Medications That Can Help to Prevent Disease

▶ *Hormones:* According to recent studies, the risks of taking the combined hormones estrogen and progestin after menopause to prevent long-term illnesses might outweigh the benefits. Talk to your doctor about whether starting or continuing to take hormones is right for you.

▶ *Breast Cancer Drugs:* If your mother, sister, or daughter has had breast cancer, talk to your doctor about the risks and benefits of taking medicines to prevent breast cancer.

Special Concern of Men

▶ *Prostate Cancer Screening:* A digital rectal exam and a PSA (prostate specific antigen) test should be done yearly beginning at age 50; African-American men, or men who have a family history of prostate cancer, should start at age 40.

What Else Can You Do to Stay Healthy?

▶ *Don't Smoke:* Talk to your doctor about quitting if you smoke. You can take medicine and get counseling to help you quit. Make a plan and set a quit date. Tell your family, friends, and coworkers that you are quitting, and ask for their support. If you are pregnant and smoke, quitting now will help both you and your baby.

▶ *Eat a Well-balanced Diet:* Eat a variety of foods, including fruit, vegetables, animal or vegetable protein (such as meat, fish, chicken, eggs, beans, lentils, or tofu), and grains (such as rice). Limit the amount of saturated fat that you eat.

▶ *Be Physically Active*: Walk, dance, ride a bike, rake leaves, or do any other physical activity you enjoy. Start small and work up to a total of 20 to 30 minutes, most days of the week.

▶ *Stay at a Healthy Weight*: Balance the number of calories you eat with the number you burn off by your activities. Remember to watch portion sizes. Talk to your doctor if you have questions about what or how much to eat.

▶ *Drink Alcohol Only in Moderation*: If you drink alcohol, one drink a day is safe for women, two drinks a day for men because of their generally larger body mass. Women who are pregnant should avoid alcohol entirely. A standard drink is one 12-ounce bottle of beer or wine cooler, one 5-ounce glass of wine, or 1.5 ounces of 80-proof distilled spirits.

11

Out and About—Managing Your Coumadin® or Warfarin Away from Home

RESTAURANTS

MOST OF US EAT at least a few meals out each week, and you might be concerned about maintaining your INR within the normal range in the face of temptation and menu selection.

Not to worry. Just be careful that the total of your daily meals remains balanced with respect to the amount of food you eat that contains vitamin K. If, like me, you eat one serving of leafy greens each day, for example, just be sure that you get it either in a meal out or at home, not both.

Be careful about sources of vitamin K that you don't usually have at home. For example, if you eat in a German restaurant and have red cabbage, don't have a salad as well. If you usually use a salad dressing that is safflower oil-based and low in vitamin K, remember that a restaurant's salad dressing might be made with a type of oil that has a higher vitamin K content, such as canola.

You don't need to obsess over these changes; small daily imbalances won't have a long-term effect.

Be careful about sources of vitamin K that you don't usually have at home.

Most importantly, remember to keep your alcohol consumption reasonable. As noted in Chapter 10, this generally means no more than one or two glasses of wine or an equivalent amount of beer or hard liquor in a day.

TRAVEL ISSUES

Unless you have other medical issues that make travel difficult, the fact that you need to take Coumadin® or warfarin should in no way deter you from traveling—on vacations wide and far, business, to see family, and all the many other reasons for getting "on the road."

You *do* need to take some simple precautions:

▶ If your trip will last for more than a few days, you might need to have your INR tested before you leave. If a trip is going to last for more than a few weeks, and depending on how consistent your INR has been previously, you might need to be tested during the trip.

▶ Be sure to pack enough medication to last the entire time you will be away. As a reminder, keep a weekly pill sorter in each of your suitcases (I learned this the hard way!).

▶ Just in case, and to be completely safe and avoid stress on an extended trip, call ahead to get the name of a pharmacy that has the brand and strength of medication you need.

▶ Keep all medications in your hand luggage, and make sure you have extra in case any travel delays occur. Do NOT put any medications that you need to take on a regular basis in your checked luggage.

▶ If you forget your medication, your hotel can be very helpful in locating an appropriate pharmacy. The pharmacist will need to get approval to provide you with the medication you need, which will probably require a call either to your pharmacy or physician—so be sure you keep those numbers handy!

▶ As noted elsewhere, be sure to wear a piece of jewelry and/or carry a card indicating you are on anticoagulant medication.

▶ Try to keep your eating habits and activity level as close to your everyday routine as possible.

▶ If you travel to areas where you need to be concerned about issues of water quality and eating raw vegetables and salads, be creative about alternatives. For example, when I was in Mexico recently, I regularly substituted guacamole for salad, which was most definitely *not* a hardship, and it followed the principle of peeling whatever can be peeled! Remember that, in many lesser developed countries, the food and water in restaurants and hotels that cater to visitors from North America and Europe is usually quite safe—look for the word "purificado" in Latin American countries.

Enjoy the trip!

Resources

A NUMBER OF WEBSITES have information about medical problems and treatments, although it can be difficult to know which ones have accurate information. The sites included here have been carefully checked for the quality of their information and recommendations.

Information provided by the National Institutes of Health, national medical societies, and other well-established organizations are reliable sources of information, although the frequency with which they are updated is variable. These include:

National Library of Medicine/
National Institutes of Health
www.nlm.nih.gov/medlineplus/healthtopics.html

National Heart, Lung, and Blood Institute
www.nhlbi.nih.gov/index.htm

National Institute of Neurological Disorders and Stroke
www.ninds.nih.gov/

Medicare
http://www.medicare.gov/

GENERAL INFORMATION

Package Inserts

The package insert for Coumadin is available on the main Coumadin® website: http://www.coumadin.com

There are currently eleven manufacturers of generic warfarin. One site that has good download information is for the Mallinkrodt generic: www.malwarfarin.com

Drug Information

Drugs.com is a wonderful resource, allowing you to search for drug indications and interactions in a variety of ways:
> http://www.drugs.com/MTM/warfarin.html

A detailed list of interactions with Coumadin and warfarin can be found at:
> http://www.drugs.com/drug-interactions/warfarin_
> d00022.html

RxList.com is an excellent site if you have questions about any medication you take:
> http://www.rxlist.com/script/main/hp.asp

Ptinr.com is a good source to check if you have questions about specific interactions:
> http://ww.ptinr.com/data/pages/section.aspx?z=3&1=full

This site is worth checking if you are prescribed a new drug:
http://www.warfarinfo.com/warfarinfo.interactions
percent20list.htm

Warfarinfo is from The Warfarin Institute of America, maintained by Al Lodwick, R.Ph., MA, a pharmacist who specialized in the monitoring and dosing of warfarin:
http://www.warfarinfo.com

Home Monitoring

Three monitors are currently available for home use: the ProTime PT/INR monitor, CoaguChek XS PST INR monitor, and the INRatio PT/INR monitor. You will need a prescription for a monitor and testing strips, and your insurance company might provide only one brand of monitor. All three can be viewed at www.ptinr.com, a site sponsored by Quality Assured Services; a Google search will provide more options for purchase should your insurance company not cover this type of "durable medical equipment."

Useful Services

The MedicAlert® Foundation, at http://www.medicalert.org, is a nonprofit organization and a repository of health information, which enables members to manage their personal health records. It provides a wide range of jewelry that every person taking Coumadin or warfarin should consider, as well as wallet cards. As a member, in an emergency, they can immediately provide needed information about your use of anticoagulants medication and the reason you are taking it.

The PT-INR Coumadin helpbook, at http://www.pt-inr.com/coumadin-helpbook, leads you to pages with a number of interactions between Coumadin or warfarin and other drugs, over-the-counter medications, foods, and more. Helpful downloads include a food diary that can be especially helpful if you are having problems maintaining your INR in the right range and are searching for a possible cause in your diet. The site is sponsored by Quality Assured Services, which specializes in home INR monitoring.

Dr. Gourmet, at www.drgourmet.com, has a sub-site from which you can download PDF files that have vitamin K content by High, Medium, and Low, or by content in micrograms (http://www.drgourmet.com/askdrgourmet/warfarin/index.shtml). For most purposes, we recommend the High, Medium, Low table, but if you are having a problem maintaining your INR in the correct range, you might find it useful to double-check the exact content of the foods you eat. This site also has helpful hints and dietary guidelines.

ActCel, BloodSTOP, and Celox are examples of "hemostatic" gauze that can be used to control emergency bleeding, such as nosebleeds or cuts. A number of websites sell these products—just Google the names for multiple sources. They are expensive, but keeping a few handy may be a good idea.

Stroke

From the National Institute of Neurologic Diseases and Stroke:
www.ninds.nih.gov/disorders/stroke/knowstroke.htm

From the American Heart Association:
www.americanheart.org/presenter.jhtml?identifier=4755

From the American Stroke Association, a division of the American Heart Association:
http://www.strokeassociation.org

From Wikipedia:
http://en.wikipedia.org/wiki/Stroke

Myocardial Infarction

From the American Heart Association:
http://www.americanheart.org/presenter.jhtml?
identifier=1200005

From the National Library of Medicine:
http://www.nlm.nih.gov/medlineplus/ency/article/
000195.htm

From Wikipedia:
http://en.wikipedia.org/wiki/Myocardial_infarction

Atrial Fibrillation

From the American Heart Association:
http://www.americanheart.org/presenter.jhtml?
identifier=4451

From the Mayo Clinic:

http://www.mayoclinic.com/health/atrial-fibrillation/
DS00291

From eMedicineHealth.com:

http://www.emedicinehealth.com/atrial_fibrillation/
article_em.htm

Pulmonary Embolism

From the Heart, Lung and Blood Institute of the National
Institutes of Health:

http://www.nhlbi.nih.gov/health/dci/Diseases/pe/
pe_what.html

From the Mayo Clinic:

http://www.mayoclinic.com/health/pulmonary-embolism/
DS00429

From eMedicineHealth.com:

http://www.emedicinehealth.com/pulmonary_embolism/
article_em.htm

Index

Note: Boldface numbers indicate illustrations; *t* indicates a table.